Alkaline Treats

Stay healthy and fit with these delicious Appetizers and
Smoothies for your Relax Moments

Isaac Vinson

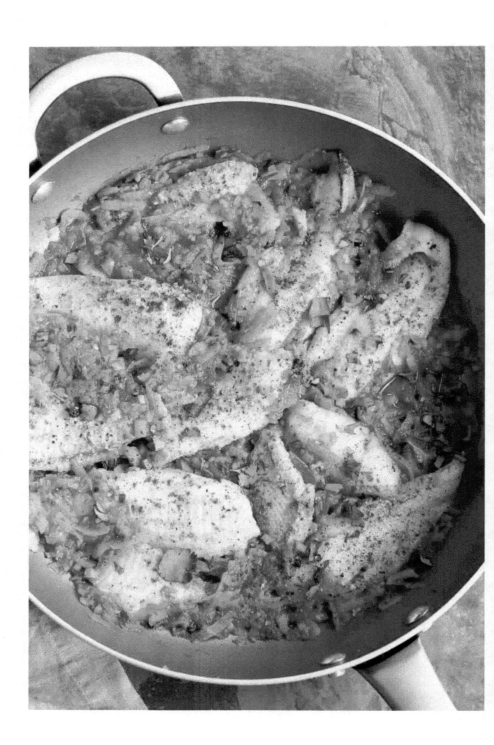

Table of Contents

4

Green Beans In Oven

Preparation Time: 5 minutes

Cooking Time: 17 minutes

Servings: 3

Ingredients

• 12 oz. green bean pods

• 1 tbsp. olive oil

• 1/2 tsp. onion powder

• 1/8 tsp. pepper

• 1/8 tsp. salt

Directions:

1. Preheat oven to 350°F. Mix green beans with onion powder, pepper, and oil.

2. Spread the seeds on the baking sheet.

3. Bake 17 minutes or until you have a delicious aroma in the kitchen.

Nutrition

37 Calories

1.4g Protein

5.5g Carbohydrates

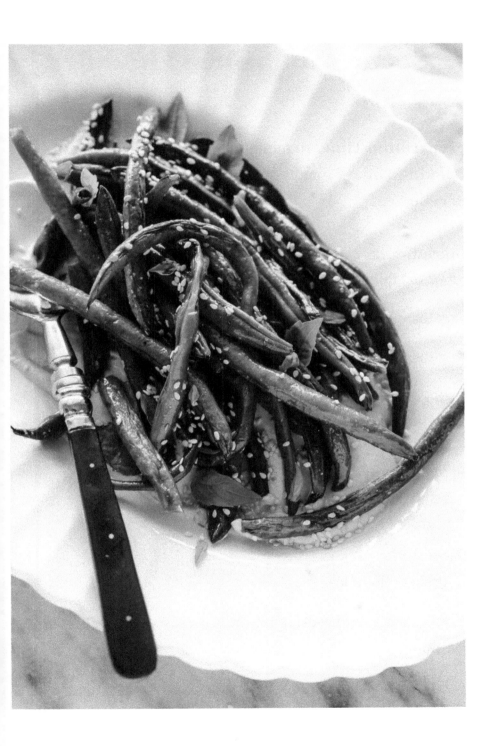

Parmesan Broiled Flounder

Preparation Time: 10 minutes

Cooking Time: 7 minutes

Servings: 2

Ingredients

• 2 (4-oz) flounder

• 1,5 tbsp Parmesan cheese

• 1,5 tbsp mayonnaise

• 1/8 tsp soy sauce

• 1/4 tsp chili sauce

• 1/8 tsp salt-free lemon-pepper seasoning

Directions:

1. Preheat flounder.

2. Mix cheese, reduced-fat mayonnaise, soy sauce, chili sauce, seasoning.

3. Put fish on a baking sheet coated with cooking spray, sprinkle with salt and pepper.

4. Spread Parmesan mixture over flounder.

5. Broil 6 to 8 minutes or until a crust appears on the fish.

Nutrition:

200 Calories

17g Fat

7g Carbohydrate

Fish With Fresh Tomato - Basil Sauce

Preparation Time: 10 minutes
Cooking Time: 15 minutes
Servings: 2

Ingredients

- 2 (4-oz) tilapia fillets

- 1 tbsp fresh basil, chopped

- 1/8 tsp salt

- 1 pinch of crushed red pepper

- 1 cup cherry tomatoes, chopped

- 2 tsp extra virgin olive oil

Directions:

1. Preheat oven to 400°F.

2. Arrange rinsed and patted dry fish fillets on foil (coat a foil baking sheet with cooking spray).

3. Sprinkle tilapia fillets with salt and red pepper.

4. Bake 12 - 15 minutes.

5. Meanwhile, mix leftover Ingredients in a saucepan.

6. Cook over medium-high heat until tomatoes are tender.

7. Top fish fillets properly with tomato mixture.

Nutrition:

130 Calories

30g Protein

1g Carbohydrates

Baked Chicken

Preparation Time: 15 minutes
Cooking Time: 25 minutes
Servings: 4

Ingredients

- 2 (6-oz) bone-in chicken breasts

- 1/8 tsp salt

- 1/8 tsp pepper

- 3 tsp extra virgin olive oil

- 1/2 tsp dried oregano

- 7 pitted kalamata olives

- 1 cup cherry tomatoes

- 1/2 cup onion

- 1 (9-oz) pkg frozen artichoke hearts

- 1 lemon

Directions:

1. Preheat oven to 400°F.

2. Sprinkle chicken with pepper, salt, and oregano.

3. Heat oil, add chicken and cook until it browned.

4. Place chicken in a baking dish. Arrange tomatoes, coarsely chopped olives, and onion, artichokes and lemon cut into wedges around the chicken.

5. Bake 20 minutes or until chicken is done and vegetables are tender.

Nutrition:

160 Calories

3g Fat

1g Carbohydrates

Seared Chicken With Roasted Vegetables

Preparation Time: 20 minutes
Cooking Time: 30 minutes
Servings: 1

Ingredients

- 1 (8-oz) boneless, skinless chicken breasts

- 3/4 lb. small Brussels sprouts

- 2 large carrots

- 1 large red bell pepper

- 1 small red onion

- 2 cloves garlic halved

- 2 tbsp extra virgin olive oil

- 1/2 tsp dried dill

- 1/4 tsp pepper

- 1/4 tsp salt

Directions:

1. Preheat oven to 425°F.

2. Match Brussels sprouts cut in half, red onion cut into wedges, sliced carrots, bell pepper cut into pieces and halved garlic on a baking sheet.

3. Sprinkle with 1 tbsp oil and with 1/8 tsp salt and 1/8 tsp pepper. Bake until well-roasted, cool slightly.

4. In the Meantime, sprinkle chicken with dill, remaining 1/8 tsp salt and 1/8 tsp pepper. Cook until chicken is done. Put roasted vegetables with drippings over chicken.

Nutrition:

170 Calories

7g Fat

12g Protein

Fish Simmered In Tomato-Pepper Sauce

Preparation Time: 5 minutes

Cooking Time: 10 minutes

Servings: 2

Ingredients

- 2 (4-oz) cod fillets

- 1 big tomato

- 1/3 cup red peppers (roasted)

- 3 tbsp almonds

- 2 cloves garlic

- 2 tbsp fresh basil leaves

- 2 tbsp extra virgin olive oil

- 1/4 tsp salt

- 1/8 tsp pepper

Directions :

1. Toast sliced almonds in a pan until fragrant.

2. Grind almonds, basil, minced garlic, 1-2 tsp oil in a food processor until finely ground.

3. Add coarsely-chopped tomato and red peppers; grind until smooth.

4. Season fish with salt and pepper.

5. Cook in hot oil in a large pan over medium-high heat until fish is browned. Pour sauce around fish. Cook 6 minutes more.

Nutrition:

90 Calories

5g Fat

7g Carbohydrates

Cheese Potato And Pea Casserole

Preparation Time: 10 minutes

Cooking Time: 35 minutes

Servings: 3

Ingredients

• 1 tbsp olive oil

• ¾ lb. red potatoes

• ¾ cup green peas

• ½ cup red onion

• ¼ tsp dried rosemary

• ¼ tsp salt

• 1/8 tsp pepper

Directions:

1. Prepare oven to 350°F.

2. Cook 1 tsp oil in a skillet. Stir in thinly sliced onions and cook. Remove from pan.

3. Situate half of the thinly sliced potatoes and onions in bottom of skillet; top with peas, crushed dried rosemary, and 1/8 tsp each salt and pepper.

4. Place remaining potatoes and onions on top. Season with remaining 1/8 tsp salt.

5. Bake 35 minutes, pour remaining 2 tsp oil and sprinkle with cheese.

Nutrition:

80 Calories

2g Protein

18g Carbohydrates

Oven-Fried Tilapia

Preparation Time: 7 minutes

Cooking Time: 15 minutes

Servings: 2

Ingredients

- 2 (4-oz) tilapia fillets

- 1/4 cup yellow cornmeal

- 2 tbsp light ranch dressing

- 1 tbsp canola oil

- 1 tsp dill (dried)

- 1/8 tsp salt

Directions:

1. Preheat oven to 425°F. Brush both sides of rinsed and patted dry tilapia fish fillets with dressing.

2. Combine cornmeal, oil, dill, and salt.

3. Sprinkle fish fillets with cornmeal mixture.

4. Put fish on a prepared baking sheet.

5. Bake 15 minutes.

Nutrition:

96 Calories

21g Protein

2g Fat

Chicken With Coconut Sauce

Preparation Time: 15 minutes

Cooking Time: 20 minutes

Servings: 2

Ingredients

- 1/2 lb. chicken breasts

- 1/3 cup red onion

- 1 tbsp paprika (smoked)

- 2 tsp cornstarch

- 1/2 cup light coconut milk

- 1 tsp extra virgin olive oil

- 2 tbsp fresh cilantro

- 1 (10-oz) can tomatoes and green chilis

- 1/4 cup water

Directions :

1. Cut chicken into little cubes; sprinkle with 1,5 tsp paprika.

2. Heat oil, add chicken and cook 3 to 5 minutes.

3. Remove from skillet, and fry finely-chopped onion 5 minutes.

4. Return chicken to pan. Add tomatoes,1,5 tsp paprika, and water. Bring to a boil, and then simmer 4 minutes.

5. Mix cornstarch and coconut milk; stir into chicken mixture, and cook until it has done.

6. Sprinkle with chopped cilantro.

Nutrition:

200 Calories

13g Protein

10g Fat

Fish With Fresh Herb Sauce

Preparation Time: 10 minutes
Cooking Time: 10 minutes
Servings: 2

Ingredients

• 2 (4-oz) cod fillets

• 1/3 cup fresh cilantro

• 1/4 tsp cumin

• 1 tbsp red onion

• 2 tsp extra virgin olive oil

• 1 tsp red wine vinegar

• 1 small clove garlic

• 1/8 tsp salt

• 1/8 black pepper

Directions:

1. Combine chopped cilantro, finely chopped onion, oil, red wine vinegar, minced garlic, and salt.

2. Sprinkle both sides of fish fillets with cumin and pepper.

3. Cook fillets 4 minutes per side. Top each fillet with cilantro mixture.

Nutrition:

90 Calories

4g Fat

3g Carbohydrates

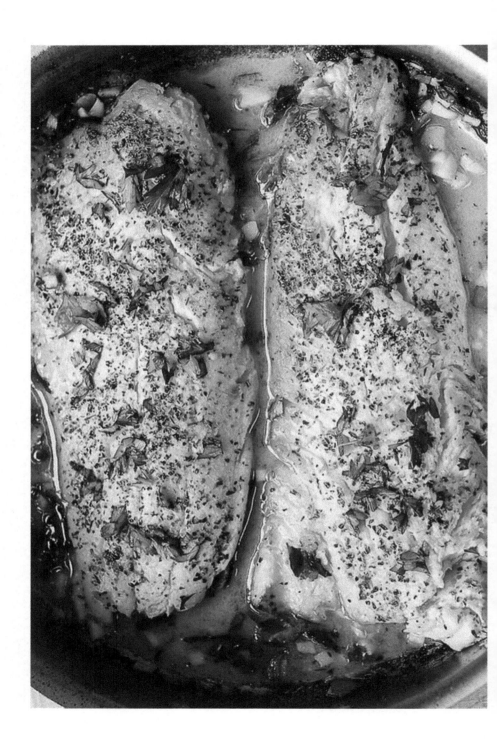

Skillet Turkey Patties

Preparation Time: 7 minutes

Cooking Time: 8 minutes

Servings: 2

Ingredients

• 1/2 lb. lean ground turkey

• 1/2 cup low-sodium chicken broth

• 1/4 cup red onion

• 1/2 tsp Worcestershire sauce

• 1 tsp extra virgin olive oil

• 1/4 tsp oregano (dried)

• 1/8 tsp pepper

Directions:

1. Combine turkey, chopped onion, Worcestershire sauce, dried oregano, and pepper; make 2 patties.

2. Warm up oil and cook patties 4 minutes per side; set aside.

3. Add broth to skillet, bring to a boil. Boil 2 minutes, spoon sauce over patties.

Nutrition:

180 Calories

11g Fat

9g Carbohydrates

Turkey Loaf

Preparation Time: 10 minutes
Cooking Time: 30 minutes
Servings: 2

Ingredients

- 1/2 lb. 93% lean ground turkey

- 1/3 cup panko breadcrumbs

- 1/2 cup green onion

- 1 egg

- 1/2 cup green bell pepper

- 1 tbsp ketchup

- 1/4 cup sauce (Picante)

- 1/2 tsp cumin (ground)

Directions:

1. Preheat oven to 350°F. Mix lean ground turkey, 3 tbsp Picante sauce, panko breadcrumbs, egg, chopped green onion, chopped green bell pepper and cumin in a bowl (mix well);

2. Put the mixture into a baking sheet; shape into an oval (about 1,5 inches thick). Bake 40 minutes.

3. Mix remaining Picante sauce and the ketchup; apply over loaf. Bake 5 minutes longer. Let stand 5 minutes.

Nutrition:

161 Calories

20g Protein

8g Fat

Mushroom Pasta

Preparation Time: 7 minutes
Cooking Time: 10 minutes
Servings: 4

Ingredients

• 4 oz whole-grain linguine

• 1 tsp extra virgin olive oil

• 1/2 cup light sauce

• 2 tbsp green onion

• 1 (8-oz) pkg mushrooms

• 1 clove garlic

• 1/8 tsp salt

• 1/8 tsp pepper

Directions:

1. Cook pasta according to package directions, drain.

2. Fry sliced mushrooms 4 minutes.

3. Stir in fettuccine minced garlic, salt and pepper. Cook 2 minutes.

4. Heat light sauce until heated; top pasta mixture properly with sauce and with finely-chopped green onion.

Nutrition:

300 Calories

1g Fat

15g Carbohydrates

Chicken Tikka Masala

Preparation Time: 5 minutes
Cooking Time: 15 minutes
Servings: 2

Ingredients

- 1/2 lb. chicken breasts

- 1/4 cup onion

- **1.** 5 tsp extra virgin olive oil

- 1 (**14.** 5-oz) can tomatoes

- 1 tsp ginger

- 1 tsp fresh lemon juice

- 1/3 cup plain Greek yogurt (fat-free)

- 1 tbsp garam masala

- 1/4 tsp salt

- 1/4 tsp pepper

Directions:

1. Flavor chicken cut into 1-inch cubes with 1,5 tsp garam masala,1/8 tsp salt and pepper.

2. Cook chicken and diced onion 4 to 5 minutes.

3. Add diced tomatoes, grated ginger, 1.5 tsp garam masala, 1/8 tsp salt. Cook 8 to 10 minutes.

4. Add lemon juice and yogurt until blended.

Nutrition:

200 Calories

26g Protein

10g Fat

Tomato And Roasted Cod

Preparation Time: 10 minutes
Cooking Time: 35 minutes
Servings: 2

Ingredients

• 2 (4-oz) cod fillets

• 1 cup cherry tomatoes

• **Servings:** cup onion

• 2 tsp orange rind

• 1 tbsp extra virgin olive oil

• 1 tsp thyme (dried)

• 1/4 tsp salt, divided

• 1/4 tsp pepper, divided

Directions:

1. Preheat oven to 400°F. Mix in half tomatoes, sliced onion, grated orange rind, extra virgin olive oil, dried thyme, and 1/8 salt and pepper. Fry 25 minutes. Remove from oven.

2. Arrange fish on pan, and flavor with remaining 1/8 tsp each salt and pepper. Put reserved tomato mixture over fish. Bake 10 minutes.

Nutrition:

120 Calories

9g Protein

2g Fat

Whole-Grain Breakfast Cookies

Preparation Time: 20 minutes

Cooking Time: 10 minutes

Servings: 18 cookies

Ingredients :

• 2 cups rolled oats

• 1/2 cup whole-wheat flour

• ¼ cup ground flaxseed

• 1 teaspoon baking powder

• 1 cup unsweetened applesauce

• 2 large eggs

• 2 tablespoons vegetable oil

• 2 teaspoons vanilla extract

• 1 teaspoon ground cinnamon

• 1/2 cup dried cherries

• ¼ cup unsweetened shredded coconut

• 2 ounces dark chocolate, chopped

Directions:

1. Preheat the oven to 350f.

2. In a large bowl, combine the oats, flour, flaxseed, and baking powder. Stir well to mix.

3. In a medium bowl, whisk the applesauce, eggs, vegetable oil, vanilla, and cinnamon. Pour the wet mixture into the dry mixture, and stir until just combined.

4. Fold in the cherries, coconut, and chocolate. Drop tablespoon-size balls of dough onto a baking sheet. Bake for 10 to 12 minutes, until browned and cooked through.

5. Let cool for about 3 minutes, remove from the baking sheet, and cool completely before serving. Store in an airtight

container for up to 1 week.

Nutrition: calories: 136;

total fat: 7g;

saturated fat: 3g;

protein: 4g;

carbs: 14g;

sugar: 4g;

fiber: 3g;

cholesterol: 21mg;

sodium: 11mg

Blueberry Breakfast Cake

Preparation Time: 15 minutes
Cooking Time: 40 minutes
Servings: 12

Ingredients :

For the topping

- ¼ cup finely chopped walnuts

- 1/2 teaspoon ground cinnamon

- 2 tablespoons butter, chopped into small pieces

- 2 tablespoons sugar

For the cake

- Nonstick cooking spray

- 1 cup whole-wheat pastry flour

- 1 cup oat flour

- ¼ cup sugar

- 2 teaspoons baking powder

- 1 large egg, beaten

- 1/2 cup skim milk

- 2 tablespoons butter, melted

- 1 teaspoon grated lemon peel

- 2 cups fresh or frozen blueberries

Directions:

To make the topping

In a small bowl, stir together the walnuts, cinnamon, butter, and sugar. Set aside.

To make the cake

1. Preheat the oven to 350f. Spray a 9-inch square pan with cooking spray. Set aside.

2. In a large bowl, stir together the pastry flour, oat flour, sugar, and baking powder.

3. Add the egg, milk, butter, and lemon peel, and stir until there are no dry spots.

4. Stir in the blueberries, and gently mix until incorporated. Press the batter into the prepared pan, using a spoon to flatten it into the dish.

5. Sprinkle the topping over the cake.

6. Bake for 40, until a toothpick inserted into the cake comes out clean, and serve.

Nutrition:

calories: 177;

total fat: 7g;

saturated fat: 3g;

protein: 4g;

carbs: 26g;

sugar: 9g;

fiber: 3g;

cholesterol: 26mg;

sodium: 39mg

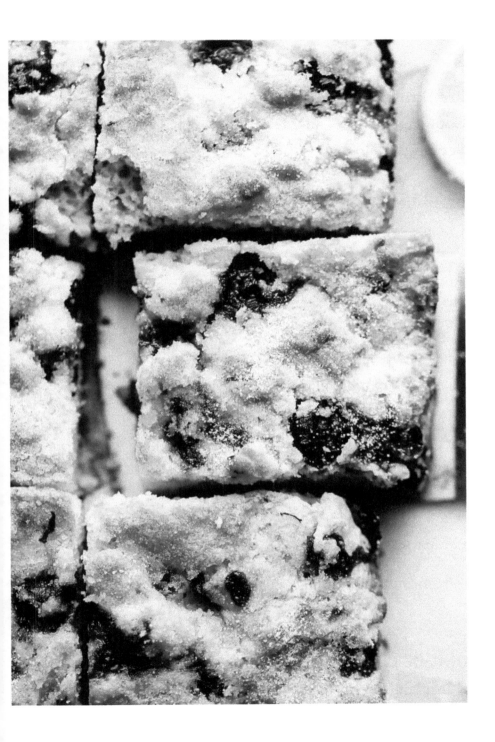

Whole-Grain Pancakes

Preparation Time: 10 minutes

Cooking Time: 15 minutes

Servings: 4 to 6

Ingredients :

• 2 cups whole-wheat pastry flour

• 4 teaspoons baking powder

• 2 teaspoons ground cinnamon

• 1/2 teaspoon salt

• 2 cups skim milk, plus more as needed

• 2 large eggs

• 1 tablespoon honey

• Nonstick cooking spray

• Maple syrup, for serving

• Fresh fruit, for serving

Directions:

1. In a large bowl, stir together the flour, baking powder, cinnamon, and salt.

2. Add the milk, eggs, and honey, and stir well to combine. If needed, add more milk, 1 tablespoon at a time, until there are no dry spots and you has a pourable batter.

3. Heat a large skillet over medium-high heat, and spray it with cooking spray.

4. Using a ¼-cup measuring cup, scoop 2 or 3 pancakes into the skillet at a time. Cook for a couple of minutes, until bubbles form on the surface of the pancakes, flip, and cook for 1 to 2 minutes more, until golden brown and cooked through. Repeat with the remaining batter.

5. Serve topped with maple syrup or fresh fruit.

Nutrition:

calories: 392;

total fat: 4g;

saturated fat: 1g;

protein: 15g;

carbs: 71g;

sugar: 11g;

fiber: 9g;

cholesterol: 95mg;

sodium: 396mg

Buckwheat Grouts Breakfast Bowl

Preparation Time: 5 minutes, plus overnight to soak

Cooking Time: 10 to 12 minutes

Servings: 4

Ingredients :

- 3 cups skim milk

- 1 cup buckwheat grouts

- ¼ cup chia seeds

- 2 teaspoons vanilla extract

- 1/2 teaspoon ground cinnamon

- Pinch salt

- 1 cup water

- 1/2 cup unsalted pistachios

- 2 cups sliced fresh strawberries

- ¼ cup cacao nibs (optional)

Directions:

1. In a large bowl, stir together the milk, groats, chia seeds, vanilla, cinnamon, and salt. Cover and refrigerate overnight.

2. The next morning, transfer the soaked mixture to a medium pot and add the water. Bring to a boil over medium-high heat, reduce the heat to maintain a simmer, and cook for 10 to 12 minutes, until the buckwheat is tender and thickened.

3. Transfer to bowls and serve, topped with the pistachios, strawberries, and cacao nibs (if using).

Nutrition:

calories: 340;

total fat: 8g;

saturated fat: 1g;

protein: 15g;

carbs: 52g;

sugar: 14g;

fiber: 10g;

cholesterol: 4mg;

sodium: 140mg

Peach Muesli Bake

Preparation Time: 10 minutes

Cooking Time: 40 minutes

Servings: 8

Ingredients :

• Nonstick cooking spray

• 2 cups skim milk

• 11/2 cups rolled oats

• 1/2 cup chopped walnuts

• 1 large egg

• 2 tablespoons maple syrup

• 1 teaspoon ground cinnamon

• 1 teaspoon baking powder

• 1/2 teaspoon salt

• 2 to 3 peaches, sliced

Directions:

1. Preheat the oven to 375f. Spray a 9-inch square baking dish with cooking spray. Set aside.

2. In a large bowl, stir together the milk, oats, walnuts, egg, maple syrup, cinnamon, baking powder, and salt. Spread half the mixture in the prepared baking dish.

3. Place half the peaches in a single layer across the oat mixture.

4. Spread the remaining oat mixture over the top. Add the remaining peaches in a thin layer over the oats. Bake for 35 to 40 minutes, uncovered, until thickened and browned.

5. Cut into 8 squares and serve warm.

Nutrition:

calories: 138;

total fat: 3g;

saturated fat: 1g;

protein: 6g;

carbs: 22g;

sugar: 10g;

fiber: 3g;

cholesterol: 24mg;

sodium: 191mg

Steel-Cut Oatmeal Bowl With Fruit And Nuts

Preparation Time: 5 minutes

Cooking Time: 20 minutes

Servings: 4

Ingredients :

• 1 cup steel-cut oats

• 2 cups almond milk

• ¾ cup water

• 1 teaspoon ground cinnamon

• ¼ teaspoon salt

• 2 cups chopped fresh fruit, such as blueberries, strawberries, raspberries, or peaches

• 1/2 cup chopped walnuts

• ¼ cup chia seeds

Directions:

1. In a medium saucepan over medium-high heat, combine the oats, almond milk, water, cinnamon, and salt. Bring to a boil, reduce the heat to low, and simmer for 15 to 20 minutes, until the oats are softened and thickened.

2. Top each bowl with 1/2 cup of fresh fruit, 2 tablespoons of walnuts, and 1 tablespoon of chia seeds before serving.

Nutrition:

calories: 288;

total fat: 11g;

saturated fat: 1g;

protein: 10g;

carbs: 38g;

sugar: 7g;

fiber: 10g;

cholesterol: 0mg;

sodium: 329mg

Whole-Grain Dutch Baby Pancake

Preparation Time: 5 minutes
Cooking Time: 25 minutes
Servings: 4

Ingredients :

- 2 tablespoons coconut oil

- 1/2 cup whole-wheat flour

- ¼ cup skim milk

- 3 large eggs

- 1 teaspoon vanilla extract

- 1/2 teaspoon baking powder

- ¼ teaspoon salt

- ¼ teaspoon ground cinnamon

- Powdered sugar, for dusting

Directions:

1. Preheat the oven to 400f.

2. Put the coconut oil in a medium oven-safe skillet, and place the skillet in the oven to melt the oil while it preheats.

3. In a blender, combine the flour, milk, eggs, vanilla, baking powder, salt, and cinnamon. Process until smooth.

4. Carefully remove the skillet from the oven and tilt to spread the oil around evenly.

5. Pour the batter into the skillet and return it to the oven for 23 to 25 minutes, until the pancake puffs and lightly browns.

6. Remove, dust lightly with powdered sugar, cut into 4 wedges, and serve.

Nutrition:

calories: 195;

total fat: 11g;

saturated fat: 7g;

protein: 8g;

carbs: 16g;

sugar: 1g;

fiber: 2g;

cholesterol: 140mg;

sodium: 209mg

Mushroom, Zucchini, And Onion Frittata

Preparation Time: 10 minutes

Cooking Time: 20 minutes

Servings: 4

Ingredients :

- 1 tablespoon extra-virgin olive oil

- 1/2 onion, chopped

- 1 medium zucchini, chopped

- 11/2 cups sliced mushrooms

- 6 large eggs, beaten

- 2 tablespoons skim milk

- Salt

- Freshly ground black pepper

- 1 ounce feta cheese, crumbled

Directions:

1. Preheat the oven to 400f.

2. In a medium oven-safe skillet over medium-high heat, heat the olive oil.

3. Add the onion and sauté for 3 to 5 minutes, until translucent.

4. Add the zucchini and mushrooms, and cook for 3 to 5 more minutes, until the vegetables are tender.

5. Meanwhile, in a small bowl, whisk the eggs, milk, salt, and pepper. Pour the mixture into the skillet, stirring to combine, and transfer the skillet to the oven. Cook for 7 to 9 minutes, until set.

6. Sprinkle with the feta cheese, and cook for 1 to 2 minutes more, until heated through.

7. Remove, cut into 4 wedges, and serve.

Nutrition:

calories: 178;

total fat: 13g;

saturated fat: 4g;

protein: 12g;

carbs: 5g;

sugar: 3g;

fiber: 1g;

cholesterol: 285mg;

sodium: 234mg

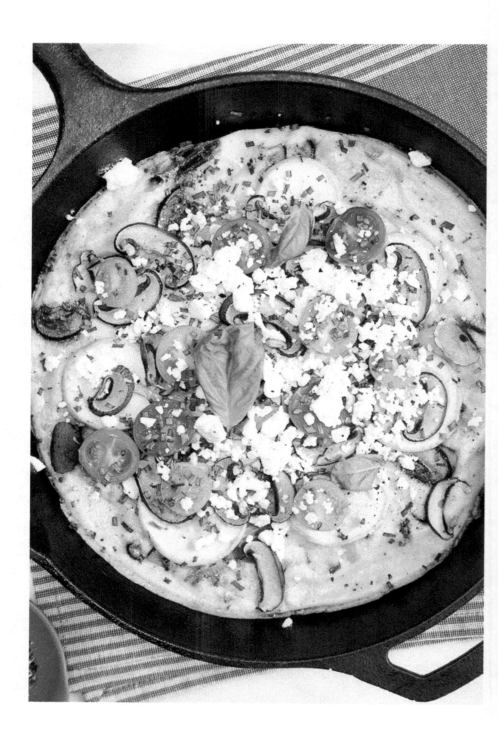

Spinach And Cheese Quiche

Preparation Time: 10 minutes, plus 10 minutes to rest

Cooking Time: 40 minutes

Servings: 4 to 6

Ingredients :

• Nonstick cooking spray

• 8 ounces yukon gold potatoes, shredded

• 1 tablespoon plus 2 teaspoons extra-virgin olive oil, divided

• 1 teaspoon salt, divided

• Freshly ground black pepper

• 1 onion, finely chopped

• 1 (10-ounce) bag fresh spinach

• 4 large eggs

• 1/2 cup skim milk

• 1 ounce gruyère cheese, shredded

Directions:

1. Preheat the oven to 350f. Spray a 9-inch pie dish with cooking spray. Set aside.

2. In a small bowl, toss the potatoes with 2 teaspoons of olive oil, 1/2 teaspoon of salt, and season with pepper. Press the potatoes into the bottom and sides of the pie dish to form a thin, even layer. Bake for 20 minutes, until golden brown. Remove from the oven and set aside to cool.

3. In a large skillet over medium-high heat, heat the remaining 1 tablespoon of olive oil.

4. Add the onion and sauté for 3 to 5 minutes, until softened.

5. By handfuls, add the spinach, stirring between each addition, until it just starts to wilt before adding more. Cook for about 1 minute, until it cooks down.

6. In a medium bowl, whisk the eggs and milk. Add the gruyère, and season with the remaining 1/2 teaspoon of salt and some pepper. Fold the eggs into the spinach. Pour the mixture into the pie dish and bake for 25 minutes, until the eggs are set.

7. Let rest for 10 minutes before serving.

Nutrition:

calories: 445;

total fat: 14g;

saturated fat: 4g;

protein: 19g;

carbs: 68g;

sugar: 6g;

fiber: 7g;

cholesterol: 193mg;

sodium: 773mg

Raisins – Plume Smoothie

Preparation Time: 10 minutes
Cooking Time: 0 minutes
Servings: 1

Ingredients :

• 1 Teaspoon Raisins

• 2 Sweet Cherry

• 1 Skinned Black Plume

• 1 Cup alkaline Stomach Calming Herbal Tea/ Cuachalate back powder,

• ¼ Coconut Water

Directions:

1. Flash 1 teaspoon of Raisin in warm water for 5 seconds and drain the water completely.

2. Rinse, cube Sweet Cherry and skinned black Plum

3. Get 1 cup of water boiled; put ¾ alkaline Stomach Calming Herbal Tea for 10 – 15minutes.

4. If you are unable to get alkaline Stomach Calming Herbal tea, you can alternatively, cook 1 teaspoon of powdered Cuachalate with 1 cup of water for 5 – 10 minutes, remove the extract and allow it to cool.

5. Pour all the ARPS items inside a blender and blend till you achieve a homogenous smoothie.

6. It is now okay, for you to enjoy the inevitable detox smoothie.

Nutrition:

Calories: 150

Fat: 1.2 g

Carbohydrates: 79 g

Protein: 3.1 g

Nori Clove Smoothies

Preparation Time: 10 minutes
Cooking Time: 0 minutes
Servings: 1

Ingredients :

- ¼ Cup Fresh Nori

- 1 Cup Cubed Banana

- 1 Teaspoon Diced Onion or ¼ Teaspoon Powdered Onion

- ½ Teaspoon Clove

- 1 Cup Alkaline Energy Booster

- 1 Tablespoon Agave Syrup

Directions:

1. Rinse ANCS Items with clean water.

2. Finely chop the onion to take one teaspoon and cut fresh Nori

3. Boil 1½ teaspoon with 2 cups of water, remove the particle, allow to cool, measure 1 cup of the tea extract

4. Pour all the items inside a blender with the tea extract and blend to achieve homogenous smoothies.

5. Transfer into a clean cup and have a nice time with a lovely body detox and energizer.

Nutrition:

Calories: 78

Fat: 2.3 g

Carbohydrates: 5 g

Protein: 6 g

Brazil Lettuce Smoothies

Preparation Time: 10 minutes
Cooking Time: 0 minutes
Servings: 1

Ingredients :

• 1 Cup Raspberries

• ½ Handful Romaine Lettuce

• ½ Cup Homemade Walnut Milk

• 2 Brazil Nuts

• ½ Large Grape with Seed

• 1 Cup Soft jelly Coconut Water

• Date Sugar to Taste

Directions:

1. In a clean bowl rinse the vegetable with clean water.

2. Chop the Romaine Lettuce and cubed Raspberries and add other items into the blender and blend to achieve homogenous smoothies.

3. Serve your delicious medicinal detox.

Nutrition:

Calories: 168

Fat: 4.5 g

Carbohydrates: 31.3 g

Sugar: 19.2 g

Protein: 3.6 g

Apple – Banana Smoothie

Preparation Time: 10 minutes

Cooking Time: 0 minutes

Servings: 1

Ingredients :

• I Cup Cubed Apple

• ½ Burro Banana

• ½ Cup Cubed Mango

• ½ Cup Cubed Watermelon

• ½ Teaspoon Powdered Onion

• 3 Tablespoon Key Lime Juice

• Date Sugar to Taste (If you like)

Directions:

1. In a clean bowl rinse the vegetable with clean water.

2. Cubed Banana, Apple, Mango, Watermelon and add other items into the blender and blend to achieve homogenous smoothies.

3. Serve your delicious medicinal detox.

4. Alternatively, you can add one tablespoon of finely dices raw red Onion if powdered Onion is not available.

Nutrition:

Calories: 99

Fat: 0.3g

Carbohydrates: 23 grams

Protein: 1.1 g

Ginger – Pear Smoothie

Preparation Time: 10 minutes

Cooking Time: 0 minutes

Servings: 1

Ingredients :

- 1 Big Pear with Seed and Cured

- ½ Avocado

- ¼ Handful Watercress

- ½ Sour Orange

- ½ Cup Ginger Tea

- ½ Cup Coconut Water

- ¼ Cup Spring Water

- 2 Tablespoon Agave Syrup

- Date Sugar to satisfaction

Directions:

1. Firstly boil 1 cup of Ginger Tea, cover the cup and allow it cool to room temperature.

2. Pour all the AGPS Items into your clean blender and homogenize them to smooth fluid.

3. You have just prepared yourself a wonderful Detox Romaine Smoothie.

Nutrition:

Calories: 101

Protein: 1 g

Carbs: 27 g

Fiber: 6 g

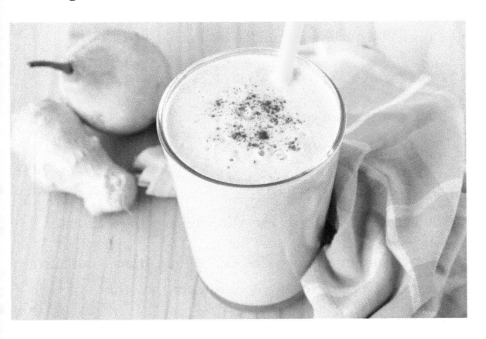

Cantaloupe – Amaranth Smoothie

Preparation Time: 10 minutes

Cooking Time: 0 minutes

Servings: 1

Ingredients :

• ½ Cup Cubed Cantaloupe

• ¼ Handful Green Amaranth

• ½ Cup Homemade Hemp Milk

• ¼ Teaspoon alkaline Bromide Plus Powder

• 1 Cup Coconut Water

• 1 Teaspoon Agave Syrup

Directions:

1. You will have to rinse all the ACAS items with clean water.

2. Chop green Amaranth, cubed Cantaloupe, transfer all into a blender and blend to achieve homogenous smoothie.

3. Pour into a clean cup; add Agave syrup and homemade Hemp Milk.

4. Stir them together and drink.

Nutrition:

Calories: 55

Fiber: 1.5 g

Carbohydrates: 8 mg

Garbanzo Squash Smoothie

Preparation Time: 10 minutes

Cooking Time: 0 minutes

Servings: 1

Ingredients :

• 1 Large Cubed Apple

• 1 Fresh Tomatoes

• 1 Tablespoon Finely Chopped Fresh Onion or ¼ Teaspoon Powdered Onion

• ¼ Cup Boiled Garbanzo Bean

• ½ Cup Coconut Milk

• ¼ Cubed Mexican Squash Chayote

• 1 Cup Energy Booster Tea

Directions:

1. You will need to rinse the AGSS items with clean water.

2. Boil 1½ Alkaline Energy Booster Tea with 2 cups of clean water. Filter the extract, measure 1 cup and allow it to cool.

3. Cook Garbanzo Bean, drain the water and allow it to cool.

4. Pour all the AGSS items into a high-speed blender and blend to achieve homogenous smoothie.

5. You may add Date Sugar.

6. Serve your amazing smoothie and drink.

Nutrition:

Calories: 82

Carbs: 22 g

Protein: 2 g

Fiber: 7 g

Strawberry – Orange Smoothies

Preparation Time: 10 minutes

Cooking Time: 0 minutes

Servings: 1

Ingredients :

• 1 Cup Diced Strawberries

• 1 Removed Back of Seville Orange

• ¼ Cup Cubed Cucumber

• ¼ Cup Romaine Lettuce

• ½ Kelp

• ½ Burro Banana

• 1 Cup Soft Jelly Coconut Water

• ½ Cup Water

• Date Sugar.

Directions:

1. Use clean water to rinse all the vegetable items of ASOS into a clean bowl.

2. Chop Romaine Lettuce; dice Strawberry, Cucumber, and Banana; remove the back of Seville Orange and divide into four.

3. Transfer all the ASOS items inside a clean blender and blend to achieve a homogenous smoothie.

4. Pour into a clean big cup and fortify your body with a palatable detox.

Nutrition:

Calories 298

Calories from Fat 9

Fat 1g

Cholesterol 2mg

Sodium 73mg

Potassium 998mg

Carbohydrates 68g

Fiber 7g

Sugar 50g

Tamarind – Pear Smoothie

Preparation Time: 10 minutes
Cooking Time: 0 minutes
Servings: 1

Ingredients :

- ½ Burro Banana

- ½ Cup Watermelon

- 1 Raspberries

- 1 Prickly Pear

- 1 Grape with Seed

- 3 Tamarind

- ½ Medium Cucumber

- 1 Cup Coconut Water

- ½ Cup Distilled Water

Directions:

1. Use clean water to rinse all the ATPS items.

2. Remove the pod of Tamarind and collect the edible part around the seed into a container.

3. If you must use the seeds then you have to boil the seed for 15mins and add to the Tamarind edible part in the container.

4. Cubed all other vegetable fruits and transfer all the items into a high-speed blender and blend to achieve homogenous smoothie.

Nutrition:

Calories: 199

Carbohydrates: 47 g

Fat: 1g

Protein: 6g

Currant Elderberry Smoothie

Preparation Time: 10 minutes

Cooking Time: 0 minutes

Servings: 1

Ingredients :

- ¼ Cup Cubed Elderberry

- 1 Sour Cherry

- 2 Currant

- 1 Cubed Burro Banana

- 1 Fig

- 1Cup 4 Bay Leaves Tea

- 1 Cup Energy Booster Tea

- Date Sugar to your satisfaction

Directions:

1. Use clean water to rinse all the ACES items

2. Initially boil ¾ Teaspoon of Energy Booster Tea with 2 cups of water on a heat source and allow boiling for 10 minutes.

3. Add 4 Bay leaves and boil together for another 4minutes.

4. Drain the Tea extract into a clean big cup and allow it to cool.

5. Transfer all the items into a high-speed blender and blend till you achieve a homogenous smoothie.

6. Pour the palatable medicinal smoothie into a clean cup and drink.

Nutrition:

Calories: 63

Fat: 0.22g

Sodium: 1.1mg

Carbohydrates: 15.5g

Fiber: 4.8g

Sugars: 8.25g

Protein: 1.6g

Sweet Dream Strawberry Smoothie

Preparation Time: 1 5 minutes

Cooking Time: 0

Servings: 1

Ingredients :

• 5 Strawberries

• 3 Dates – Pits eliminated

• 2 Burro Bananas or small bananas

• Spring Water for 32 fluid ounce of smoothie

Directions:

1. Strip off skin of the bananas.

2. Wash the dates and strawberries.

3. Include bananas, dates, and strawberries to a blender container.

4. Include a couple of water and blend.

5. Keep on including adequate water to persuade up to be 32 oz. of smoothie.

Nutrition:

Calories: 282

Fat: 11g

Carbohydrates: 4g

Protein: 7g

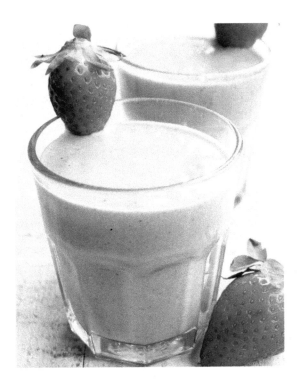

Alkaline Green Ginger And Banana Cleansing Smoothie

Preparation Time: 15 minutes

Cooking Time: 0

Servings: 1

Ingredients :

• One handful of kale

• one banana, frozen

• Two cups of hemp seed milk

• One inch of ginger, finely minced

• Half cup of chopped strawberries, frozen

• 1 tablespoon of agave or your preferred sweetener

Directions:

1. Mix all the Ingredients in a blender and mix on high speed.

2. Allow it to blend evenly.

3. Pour into a pitcher with a few decorative straws and voila you are one happy camper.

4. Enjoy!

Nutrition:

Calories: 350

Fat: 4g

Carbohydrates: 52g

Protein: 16g

Orange Mixed Detox Smoothie

Preparation Time: 15 minutes

Cooking Time: 0

Servings: 1

Ingredients :

• One cup of vegies (Amaranth, Dandelion, Lettuce or Watercress)

• Half avocado

• One cup of tender-jelly coconut water

• One seville orange

• Juice of one key lime

• One tablespoon of bromide plus powder

Directions:

1. Peel and cut the Seville orange in chunks.

2. Mix all the Ingredients collectively in a high-speed blender until done.

Nutrition:

Calories: 71

Fat: 1g

Carbohydrates: 12g

Protein: 2g

Cucumber Toxin Flush Smoothie

Preparation Time: 15 minutes

Cooking Time: 0

Servings: 1

Ingredients :

• 1 Cucumber

• 1 Key Lime

• 1 cup of watermelon (seeded), cubed

Directions:

1. Mix all the above Ingredients in a high-speed blender.

2. Considering that watermelon and cucumbers are largely water, you may not want to add any extra, however you can so if you want.

3. Juice the key lime and add into your smoothie.

4. Enjoy!

Nutrition:

Calories: 219

Fat: 4g

Carbohydrates: 48g

Protein: 5g

Apple Blueberry Smoothie

Preparation Time: 15 minutes

Cooking Time: 0

Servings: 1

Ingredients :

• Half apple

• One Date

• Half cup of blueberries

• Half cup of sparkling callaloo

• One tablespoon of hemp seeds

• One tablespoon of sesame seeds

• Two cups of sparkling soft-jelly coconut water

• Half of tablespoon of bromide plus powder

Directions:

Mix all of the Ingredients in a high-speed blender and enjoy!

Nutrition:

Calories: 167.4

Fat: 6.4g

Carbohydrates: 22.5g

Protein: 6.7g

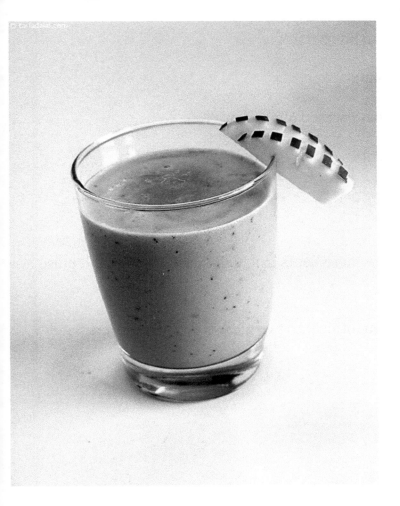

Blueberry Smoothie

Preparation Time: 10 minutes

Cooking Time: 0 minutes

Servings: 2

Ingredients :

- 2 cups frozen blueberries

- 1 small banana

- 1½ cups unsweetened almond milk

- ¼ cup ice cubes

Directions:

1. Place all the Ingredients in a high-speed blender and pulse until creamy.

2. Pour the smoothie into two glasses and serve immediately.

Nutrition:

Calories 158

Total Fat 3.3 g

Saturated Fat 0.3 g

Cholesterol 0 mg

Sodium 137 mg

Total Carbs 34 g

Fiber 5.6 g

Sugar 20.6 g

Protein 2.4 g

Beet & Strawberry Smoothie

Preparation Time: 10 minutes

Cooking Time: 0 minutes

Servings: 2

Ingredients :

• 2 cups frozen strawberries, pitted and chopped

• **Servings:** cup roasted and frozen beet, chopped

• 1 teaspoon fresh ginger, peeled and grated

• 1 teaspoon fresh turmeric, peeled and grated

• ½ cup fresh orange juice

• 1 cup unsweetened almond milk

Directions:

1. Place all the Ingredients in a high-speed blender and pulse until creamy.

2. Pour the smoothie into two glasses and serve immediately.

Nutrition:

Calories 258

Total Fat 1.5 g

Saturated Fat 0.1 g

Cholesterol 0 mg

Sodium 134 mg

Total Carbs 26.7g

Fiber 4.9 g

Sugar 18.7 g

Protein 2.9 g

Kiwi Smoothie

Preparation Time: 10 minutes

Cooking Time: 0 minutes

Servings: 2

Ingredients :

• 4 kiwis

• 2 small bananas, peeled

• 1½ cups unsweetened almond milk

• 1-2 drops liquid stevia

• ¼ cup ice cubes

Directions:

1. Place all the Ingredients in a high-speed blender and pulse until creamy.

2. Pour the smoothie into two glasses and serve immediately.

Nutrition:

Calories 228

Total Fat 3.8 g

Saturated Fat 0.4 g

Cholesterol 0 mg

Sodium 141 mg

Total Carbs 50.7 g

Fiber 8.4 g

Sugar 28.1 g

Protein 3.8 g

Pineapple & Carrot Smoothie

Preparation Time: 10 minutes

Cooking Time: 0 minutes

Servings: 2

Ingredients :

- 1 cup frozen pineapple

- 1 large ripe banana, peeled and sliced

- ½ tablespoon fresh ginger, peeled and chopped

- ¼ teaspoon ground turmeric

- 1 cup unsweetened almond milk

- ½ cup fresh carrot juice

- 1 tablespoon fresh lemon juice

Directions:

1. Place all the Ingredients in a high-speed blender and pulse until creamy.

2. Pour the smoothie into two glasses and serve immediately.

Nutrition:

Calories 132

Total Fat 2.2 g

Saturated Fat 0.3 g

Cholesterol 0 mg

Sodium 113 mg

Total Carbs 629.3 g

Fiber 4.1 g

Sugar 16.9 g

Protein 2 g

Oats & Orange Smoothie

Preparation Time: 10 minutes

Cooking Time: 0 minutes

Servings: 4

Ingredients :

• Servings: cup rolled oats

• 2 oranges, peeled, seeded, and sectioned

• 2 large bananas, peeled and sliced

• 2 cups unsweetened almond milk

• 1 cup ice cubes, crushed

Directions:

1. Place all the Ingredients in a high-speed blender and pulse until creamy.

2. Pour the smoothie into four glasses and serve immediately.

Nutrition:

Calories 175

Total Fat 3 g

Saturated Fat 0.4 g

Cholesterol 0 mg

Sodium 93 mg

Total Carbs 36.6 g

Fiber 5.9 g

Sugar 17.1 g

Protein 3.9 g

Pumpkin Creamed Smoothie

Preparation Time: 10 minutes

Cooking Time: 0 minutes

Servings: 2

Ingredients :

- 1 cup homemade pumpkin puree

- 1 medium banana, peeled and sliced

- 1 tablespoon maple syrup

- 1 teaspoon ground flaxseeds

- ½ teaspoon ground cinnamon

- ¼ teaspoon ground ginger

- 1½ cups unsweetened almond milk

- ¼ cup ice cubes

Directions:

1. Place all the Ingredients in a high-speed blender and pulse until creamy.

2. Pour the smoothie into two glasses and serve immediately.

Nutrition:

Calories 159

Total Fat 3.6 g

Saturated Fat 0.5 g

Cholesterol 0 mg

Sodium 143 mg

Total Carbs 32.6 g

Fiber 6.5 g

Sugar 17.3 g

Protein 3 g

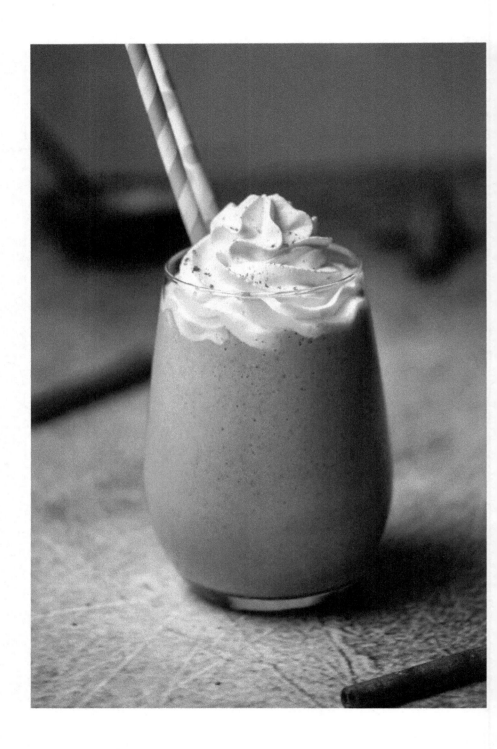